Study Guide to Accompany

Foundations of Maternal & Pediatric Nursing
Second Edition

Study Guide to Accompany

Foundations of Maternal & Pediatric Nursing

Second Edition

Lois White, RN, PhD

Former Chairperson and Professor
Department of Vocational Nurse Education
Del Mar College
Corpus Christi, Texas

Prepared by
Brandy Coward, BSN
Director of Nursing
Career Networks Institute

Previous edition prepared by
Kathleen Peck Schaefer, RNC, MSN, MEd

THOMSON

DELMAR LEARNING Australia Canada Mexico Singapore Spain United Kingdom United States

THOMSON

DELMAR LEARNING

Study Guide to Accompany Foundations of Maternal & Pediatric Nursing, Second Edition
by Lois White, RN, PhD
Prepared by Brandy Coward

Vice President,
  Health Care Business Unit:
William Brottmiller
Editorial Director:
Cathy L. Esperti
Acquisitions Editor:
Melissa Martin
Senior Developmental Editor:
Elisabeth F. Williams
Editorial Assistant:
Patricia Osborn

Marketing Director:
Jennifer McAvey
Marketing Coordinator:
Karen Summerlin
Production Director:
Karen Leet
Production Manager:
Barbara A. Bullock

Project Editor:
Natalie Wager
Art/Design Specialist:
Jay Purcell
Production Editor:
John Mickelbank
Technology Project Manager:
Victoria Moore
Technology Production Coordinator:
Sherry Conners

Library of Congress Catalog Number:
2004012414

ISBN 1-4018-2700-4

International Divisions List

Asia (including India):
Thomson Learning
60 Albert Street, #15-01
Albert Complex
Singapore 189969
Tel 65 336-6411
Fax 65 336-7411

Australia/New Zealand:
Nelson
102 Dodds Street
South Melbourne
Victoria 3205
Australia
Tel 61 (0)3 9685-4111
Fax 61 (0)3 9685-4199

Latin America:
Thomson Learning
Seneca 53
Colonia Polanco
11560 Mexico, D.F. Mexico
Tel (525) 281-2906
Fax (525) 281-2656

Canada:
Nelson
1120 Birchmount Road
Toronto, Ontario
Canada M1K 5G4
Tel (416) 752-9100
Fax (416) 752-8102

UK/Europe/Middle East/Africa:
Thomson Learning
Berkshire House
1680-173 High Holborn
London WC1V 7AA
United Kingdom
Tel 44 (0)20 497-1422
Fax 44 (0)20 497-1426

Spain (including Portugal):
Paraninfo
Calle Magallanes 25
28015 Madrid
España
Tel 34 (0)91 446-3350
Fax 34 (0)91 445-6218

Notice to the Reader

Publisher does not warrant or guarantee any of the products described herein or perform any independent analysis in connection with any of the product information contained herein. Publisher does not assume, and expressly disclaims, any obligation to obtain and include information other than that provided to it by the manufacturer.

The reader is expressly warned to consider and adopt all safety precautions that might be indicated by the activities described herein and to avoid all potential hazards. By following the instructions contained herein, the reader willingly assumes all risks in connection with such instructions.

The publisher makes no representations or warranties of any kind, including but not limited to, the warranties of fitness for particular purpose or merchantability, nor are any such representations implied with respect to the material set forth herein, and the publisher takes no responsibility with respect to such material. The publisher shall not be liable for any special, consequential, or exemplary damages resulting, in whole or part, from the reader's use of, or reliance upon, this material.

Contents

Preface . . . . *vii*

Acknowledgments. . . . . *ix*

UNIT 1: NURSING CARE OF THE CLIENT: CHILDBEARING

1 Prenatal Care 1

2 Complications of Pregnancy 9

3 The Birth Process 17

4 Postpartum Care................................27

5 Newborn Care 35

UNIT 2: NURSING CARE OF THE CLIENT: CHILDREARING

6 Basics of Pediatric Care 43

7 Infants with Special Needs: Birth to 12 months 49

8 Common Problems: 1–18 years............55

ANSWER KEY 61

Preface

This Study Guide is designed to accompany *Foundations of Maternal & Pediatric Nursing,* Second Edition, by Lois White. Each of the eight chapters in this guide was created to facilitate student learning and refine student skills. By using this guide at home and in the clinical setting you will work with important concepts and begin to apply them to real-life situations.

To facilitate your learning, each chapter in this guide includes the following components:

- *Key Terms Review*: a matching exercise designed to enhance your understanding of new terms presented in the text.
- *Abbreviation Review*: exercise to test your knowlege of abbreviations, acronyms, and symbols used in the text.
- *Exercises and Activities*: short scenarios with related questions to test your understanding and application of concepts.
- *Self-Assessment Questions*: multiple-choice questions that draw on the key ideas in the chapter and prepare you to succeed in your examinations.

Acknowledgments

I would like to thank my husband, Scott, and my children, Veronika and Trevor, for their encouragement and support. I would also like to thank the Thomson Delmar Learning team, especially Patricia Osborn and Elisabeth Williams, for their guidance and motivation.

Prenatal Care

Key Terms

Match the following terms with their correct definitions.

_____ 1. Abortion

_____ 2. Age of viability

_____ 3. Amenorrhea

_____ 4. Amnion

_____ 5. Anticipatory guidance

_____ 6. Ballottement

_____ 7. Blastocyst

_____ 8. Braxton-Hicks contractions

_____ 9. Chadwick's sign

_____10. Chloasma

_____11. Chorion

_____12. Coitus

_____13. Colostrum

_____14. Copulation

_____15. Cotyledon

_____16. Couvade

_____17. Decidua

_____18. Ductus arteriosus

a. Delivery after 24 weeks' gestation but before 38 weeks (full term).

b. False pregnancy.

c. Sexual act that delivers sperm to the cervix by ejaculation of the erect penis.

d. Gestational age at which a fetus could live outside the uterus, generally considered to be 24 weeks.

e. Descriptor for a pregnancy between 38 and 42 weeks' gestation.

f. Rebounding of the floating fetus when pushed upward though the vagina or abdomen.

g. Fetal vessel connecting the pulmonary trunk to the aorta.

h. Structure that connects the fetus to the placenta.

i. Absence of menses.

j. Loss of pregnancy before the age of viability, usually considered to be 24 weeks.

k. White, creamy substance covering the fetus's body.

l. Information, teaching, and guidance given to a client in anticipation of an expected event.

m. Darkening of the skin of the forehead and around the eyes; also called "mask of pregnancy."

n. Fecal material stored in the fetal intestines.

o. Practice of eating substances not considered edible and that have no nutritive value such as laundry starch, dirt, clay, and freezer frost.

p. Delivery after 42 weeks' gestation.

q. Fertilized ovum.

r. Condition of being pregnant for the first time.

___19. Ductus venosus

___20. Fertilization

___21. Foramen ovale

___22. Fundus

___23. Funic souffle

___24. Goodell's sign

___25. GP/TPAL

___26. Gravida

___27. Hegar's sign

___28. Implantation

___29. Lanugo

___30. Leopold's maneuvers

___31. Linea nigra

___32. Meconium

___33. Morula

___34. Multigravida

___35. Multipara

___36. Nesting

___37. Nulligrava

___38. Nullipara

___39. Para

s. Lowering of blood pressure in a pregnant woman when lying supine due to compression of the vena cava by the enlarged, heavy uterus.

t. Inner fetal membrane originating in the blastocyst.

u. Sexual act that delivers sperm to the cervix by ejaculation of the erect penis.

v. Flap opening in the atrial septum that allows only right to left movement of blood.

w. Condition of having delivered once after 24 weeks' gestation.

x. Thick substance surrounding and protecting the vessels of the umbilical cord.

y. Care of a woman during pregnancy, before labor.

z. Outer fetal membrane formed from the trophoblast.

aa. Irregular, painless uterine contractions felt by the pregnant woman toward the end of pregnancy.

bb. Mental and physical preparation for childbirth; synonymous with Lamaze.

cc. Purplish blue color of the cervix and vagina noted at about week 8 of pregnancy.

dd. Development of physical symptoms by the expectant father such as fatigue, depression, headache, backache, and nausea.

ee. Pregnancy, regardless of duration, including present pregnancy.

ff. Descriptor for when the mother feels the fetus move, about 16 to 20 weeks' gestation.

gg. The mammalian conceptus in the postmorula stage.

hh. Hemodilution caused by the increased maternal blood volume.

ii. Membranous vascular organ connecting the fetus to the mother, which produces hormones to sustain a pregnancy, supplies the fetus with oxygen and food, and transports waste products out of the fetal system.

jj. Reddish streaks frequently found on the abdomen, thighs, buttocks, and breasts; also called stretch marks.

kk. Series of specific palpations of the pregnant uterus to determine fetal position and presentation.

ll. Top of the uterus.

mm. Dark line on the abdomen from umbilicus to symphysis during pregnancy.

___40. Physiologic anemia
of pregnancy

nn. Agent such as radiation, drugs, viruses, and other micro-organisms capable of causing abnormal fetal development.

___41. Pica

oo. Sound of blood pulsating through the uterus and placenta.

___42. Placenta

pp. Condition of being pregnant two or more times.

___43. Post-term

qq. Branch of the umbilical vein that enters the inferior vena cava.

___44. Prenatal care

rr. Condition of having delivered twice or more after 24 weeks' gestation.

___45. Preterm

ss. Embedding of a fertilized egg into the uterine lining.

___46. Primigravida

tt. Antibody-rich yellow fluid secreted by the breasts during the last trimester of pregnancy and first 2 to 3 days after birth; gradually changes to milk.

___47. Primipara

uu. Fine hair covering the fetus's body.

___48. Pseudocyesis

vv. Softening of the cervix noted about week 8 of pregnancy.

___49. Psychoprophylaxis

ww. Condition of never having been pregnant.

___50. Quickening

xx. Softening of the uterine isthmus about week 6 of pregnancy.

___51. Striae gravidarum

yy. Gravida, para/term, preterm, abortions, living.

___52. Supine hypotensive
syndrome

zz. Condition of having delivered (given birth) after 24 weeks' gestation, regardless of whether infant is born alive or dead or number of infants born.

___53. Teratogen

aaa. Subdivision on the maternal side of the placenta.

___54. Term

bbb. Union of an ovum and a sperm.

___55. Umbilical cord

ccc. Sound of blood pulsating through the umbilical cord; rate the same as the fetal heartbeat.

___56. Uterine souffle

ddd. Surge of energy late in pregnancy when the pregnant woman organizes and cleans the house.

___57. Vernix caseosa

eee. Condition of never having delivered an infant after 24 weeks' gestation.

___58. Wharton's jelly

fff. The endometrium after implantation of the trophoblast.

___59. Zygote

ggg. A solid mass of cells formed by cleavage of a zygote.

Abbreviation Review

Write the meaning or definition of the following abbreviations, acronyms, and symbols.

1. ASPO _____

2. AWHONN _____

3. BOW _____

4. BPD _____

5. C-H _____

6. C-R _____

7. DES _____

8. EDB _____

9. EDD _____

10. GP/TPAL _____

11. GFR _____

12. hCG _____

13. Hgb F _____

14. hPL _____

15. ICEA _____

16. LMP _____

17. NAACOG _____

18. OTC _____

19. PBI _____

Exercises and Activities

1. What is the importance of prenatal care for the woman and her baby?

    _____

    _____

    _____

    _____

2. List several factors that can affect the development of the fetus.

    (1) _____   (5) _____

    (2) _____   (6) _____

    (3) _____   (7) _____

    (4) _____   (8) _____

3. Your client is a 23-year-old with insulin-dependent diabetes who is hoping to become pregnant within the next year. Why is it important for her to begin preconception care now?

    _____

    _____

    _____

4. Describe the physiological changes and symptoms that occur with pregnancy in the following systems.

    Cardiovascular: _____

    _____

    Respiratory: _____

    _____

    Musculoskeletal: _____

    _____

Gastrointestinal: _____

_____

Urinary: _____

_____

5. Draw a line under each of the "probable" signs of pregnancy, and draw a circle around those that are "positive" signs.

Amenorrhea	Abdominal enlargement	Chadwick's sign
Funic souffle	Breast tenderness	Braxton-Hicks contractions
Fatigue	Goodell's sign	Fetus visualization
Quickening	Uterine enlargement	Uterine souffle
Ballottement	Chloasma	Hegar's sign
Positive pregnancy test	Morning sickness	Linea nigra
Fetal heartbeat	Fetal movement by examiner	

6. List four developmental tasks of pregnancy.

(1) _____

(2) _____

(3) _____

(4) _____

7. How does the father or support person prepare for the birth of the baby?

_____

_____

8. What causes each of these common discomforts? Identify two or more interventions that can help to relieve each one.

	Cause	Interventions
Nausea/vomiting		
Constipation		
Ankle edema		
Dyspnea		
Leg cramps		
Dizziness/fainting		

9. Fatima is a 29-year-old mother of two children, ages 3 and 7, and is now 34 weeks pregnant. Fatima tells you that she wants to do everything she can to prepare her children for the birth of their new baby brother or sister. What suggestions can you give her?

_____

_____

_____

10. The nurse asks you to review the warning signs for hypertension/preeclampsia with Fatima before she leaves today. What information will you include?

   _____

   _____

11. Convert each of the following to the abbreviated form (G_P_/T_P_A_L_) for these clients.

   (1) _____ Second pregnancy, one child at home who was born at 38 weeks

   (2) _____ First pregnancy (now at 22 weeks)

   (3) _____ Pregnant for the third time; the first pregnancy ended in a miscarriage at 11 weeks; the second ended with a full-term birth; one living child at home

   (4) _____ Nulligravida

   (5) _____ Second pregnancy with twins; first pregnancy resulted in twins born at 34 weeks, who are doing well

12. Using Naegele's rule, calculate the EDB for each of the following:

LMP July 9	EDB _____
LMP December 22	EDB _____
LMP February 1	EDB _____
LMP May 15	EDB _____

13. Sarah is a 23-year-old child-care worker who is pregnant for the second time. She tells you that her first child, a 3-year-old boy, was born prematurely at 34 weeks but is doing well now. Sarah says that she was so young when she had her first baby that she didn't feel ready. She had no prenatal care until late in the pregnancy. Sarah would have preferred to become pregnant next year rather than now. However, this time she really wants to take care of herself and have a full-term, healthy baby.

   a. You write on the prenatal assessment form that Sarah is G__P__/T__P__A__L__.
   The date of her LMP was June 12, so you note that her EDB is _____.

   b. Sarah appears to be completing the first developmental task of pregnancy because:

   _____

   _____

   c. Sarah is about nine weeks pregnant now. When you ask about any discomforts that she may be experiencing, she tells you that she is having some heartburn and mood swings. You advise her to:

   _____

   _____

   d. Besides a thorough health history, what else will the first visit include?

   _____

   _____

   e. Sarah has a few questions for you. Can you help?
   "How soon can you hear the baby's heartbeat?" _____

"How big is the baby right now?" _____

"When will I feel the baby move?" _____

"How often do I have to come to the clinic?" _____

"I want to know if it's a boy or a girl. Can I get an ultrasound to find out?" _____

f. Sarah returns for one of her follow-up prenatal visits when she is 28 weeks pregnant.

What would you expect for a fundal height measurement at this time? _____

What is the approximate weight gain you would expect by this time? _____

What other tests will probably be done at this visit?

_____

_____

g. You mention the childbirth classes your hospital offers. Sarah says, "I've been through this once already, so I don't see how going to classes would really help me. Nothing helps labor, anyway." What would you tell her about the benefits of attending a prepared childbirth class?

_____

_____

_____

_____

_____

_____

Self-Assessment Questions

Circle the letter that corresponds to the best answer.

1. The nurse measuring the fundal height of a client who is 20 weeks pregnant finds it at the level of her umbilicus. The nurse determines that this
   a. is a normal finding.
   b. is greater than expected.
   c. indicates oligohydramnios.
   d. requires an immediate ultrasound.

2. You review lab work on your client, who is 32 weeks pregnant. You note that she has a hematocrit of 34%. This is most likely caused by
   a. iron deficiency anemia.
   b. poor dietary intake of protein.
   c. placental transport of blood to the fetus.
   d. hemodilution from an increase in plasma.

3. When the client complains about the Braxton-Hicks contractions she is experiencing, the nurse explains that their purpose is to
   a. soften and dilate the cervix.
   b. help her to practice breathing techniques.
   c. help with uterine and placental circulation.
   d. improve the abdominal muscle tone for delivery.

4. A client has gone into labor at 23 weeks of gestation. The nurse understands that this is below the age of viability for the infant because
   a. there is an absent suck/swallow reflex.
   b. alveoli are insufficient for air exchange.
   c. the infant has fetal hemoglobin present.
   d. the fetus has passed meconium in utero.

5. A client in the prenatal clinic is scheduled to have the following tests during her pregnancy. Which of these would be used to screen for possible birth defects?
   a. Venereal Disease Research Laboratory
   b. Rubella titer
   c. Coomb's test
   d. Alpha-fetoprotein

6. A nurse is reviewing data for her client, a 37-year-old primigravida who is now at 35 weeks' gestation. Her blood pressure today is 150/85, and she is complaining of mild edema in her legs. You determine that according to her usual blood pressure of 120/68, this is
   a. high and needs to be reported.
   b. a typical increase in the last month of pregnancy.
   c. abnormal only if the client also has edema in her hands and face.
   d. a result of a later maternal age in an otherwise normal pregnancy.

7. Fathers who smoke and mothers who do not
   a. have lower-birth-weight infants.
   b. have infants who are unaffected.
   c. have large-for-gestational age infants.
   d. have normal-weight infants.

8. The trophoblast secretes _____ during the early pregnancy.
   a. estrogen
   b. progesterone
   c. hPL
   d. hCG

9. The fetal stage of development from the beginning of week 3 through week 8 is called
   a. germinal stage.
   b. embryonic stage.
   c. fetal stage.
   d. cephalo stage.

10. At what week of fetal development is lanugo only on the shoulders and upper back?
    a. Week 28
    b. Week 32
    c. Week 36
    d. Week 40

Complications of Pregnancy

Key Terms

Match the following terms with their correct definitions.

___ 1. Abortion

___ 2. Abruptio placenta

___ 3. Amniocentesis

___ 4. Early deceleration

___ 5. Eclampsia

___ 6. Ectopic pregnancy

___ 7. Euglycemia

___ 8. Fetal biophysical profile

___ 9. HELLP syndrome

___10. Hydatidiform mole

___11. Hydramnios

___12. Hyperemesis gravidarum

___13. Incompetent cervix

___14. Kernicterus

a. Pregnancy in which the fertilized ovum is implanted outside the uterine cavity.

b. Reduction in fetal heart rate that begins after the uterus has begun contraction and increases to the baseline level after the uterine contraction has ceased.

c. Assessment of five variables: fetal breathing movement, fetal movements of body or limbs, fetal tone (flexion/extension of extremities), amniotic fluid volume, and reactive NST.

d. Termination of a pregnancy before viability of the fetus, usually 24 weeks.

e. Withdrawal of amniotic fluid to obtain a sample for specimen examination.

f. Abnormality of the placenta wherein the chorionic villi become fluid-filled, grapelike clusters; the trophoblastic tissue proliferates; and there is no viable fetus.

g. Deficiency in the amount of amniotic fluid.

h. Reduction in fetal heart rate that begins early with the contraction and virtually mirrors the uterine contraction.

i. Excessive fetal growth characterized by a fetus weighing more than 4,000 g (8.8 lb).

j. Reduction in fetal heart rate that has no relationship to contractions of the uterus.

k. Normal blood glucose level.

l. Premature separation, from the wall of the uterus, of normally implanted placenta.

m. Convulsion occurring in pregnancy-induced hypertension.

n. Pregnancy-induced hypertension with liver damage characterized by hemolysis, elevated liver enzymes, and low platelet count.

___15. Late deceleration

___16. Macrosomia

___17. Miscarriage

___18. Oligohydramnios

___19. Placenta Previa

___20. Preeclampsia

___21. Tocolysis

___22. Variable deceleration

o. Spontaneous abortion.

p. Excessive vomiting during pregnancy.

q. Condition in which the placenta forms over or very near the internal cervicalos.

r. Excess amount of amniotic fluid.

s. Descriptor for when the cervix begins to dilate, usually during the second trimester.

t. Phase of pregnancy-induced hypertension prior to convulsions.

u. Severe neurological damage resulting from a high level of bilirubin (jaundice).

v. Process of stopping labor with medications.

Abbreviation Review

Write the meaning or definition of the following abbreviations, acronyms, and symbols.

1. CMV _____

2. CST _____

3. CVS _____

4. D&C _____

5. DIC _____

6. EDB _____

7. EFM _____

8. FAST _____

9. FBPP _____

10. FHR _____

11. FHT _____

12. GDM _____

13. hCG _____

14. HELLP _____

15. hPL _____

16. HSV-2 _____

17. IUGR _____

18. L/S _____

19. $MgSO_4$ _____

20. MSAFP _____

21. NST _____

22. PG _____

23. PIH _____

24. PKU _____

25. RhoGam _____

26. SGA _____

27. TORCH _____

28. VST _____

Exercises and Activities

1. What role does fetal assessment play during pregnancy?

   _____

   _____

2. If a pregnancy is determined to be high-risk, what monitoring may be used to assess fetal well-being?

   _____

   _____

3. List several abnormal conditions that can be detected with ultrasound.

   (1) _____   (4) _____

   (2) _____   (5) _____

   (3) _____   (6) _____

4. Describe a "normal" finding for a nonstress test.

   _____

   _____

5. Describe a "normal" finding for a contraction stress test.

   _____

   _____

   _____

6. Identify the variables that are assessed with a biophysical profile.

   (1) _____

   (2) _____

   (3) _____

   (4) _____

   (5) _____

7. What information is obtained with each of the following tests? What is the expected change in laboratory values as the pregnancy progresses?

   MSAFP:_____

   Estriol:_____

   hPL:_____

   L/S ratio:_____

8. Marissa is identified as being high-risk with her current pregnancy because her last pregnancy resulted in a fetal demise 2 years ago. She has been advised to check fetal activity daily at home. How will you instruct Marissa to use the Cardiff method to monitor fetal well-being? Include warning signs.

   _____

   _____

   _____

9. Ji-Yoon, who is 32 weeks pregnant, was involved in an automobile accident. You will be assessing her for fetal well-being. What are the advantages of external fetal monitoring for this client?

   _____

   _____

   _____

10. Stephanie is a 39-year-old, G2 P1, being seen for her first prenatal visit. She is concerned about possible genetic problems with this pregnancy because of her age and a family history of birth defects. What tests could be done to reassure Stephanie? When could each test be done?

    _____

    _____

    _____

11. Briefly describe the signs and symptoms and the medical–surgical management for the following obstetrical disorders.

	Signs/Symptoms	*Medical–Surgical Management*
Incompetent cervix		
Ectopic pregnancy		
Hydatidiform mole		

   a. What follow-up care is important to the client with hydatidiform mole?

   _____

   _____

   b. How would you explain the difference between placenta previa and abruptio placenta?

   _____

   _____

   c. List several obstetrical disorders that can lead to DIC.

   (1) _____   (5) _____

   (2) _____   (6) _____

   (3) _____   (7) _____

   (4) _____

d. How can abruptio placenta lead to DIC?

_____

_____

e. What effect can each of the following disorders have on the fetus?

Maternal PKU: _____

Rubella: _____

CMV: _____

Herpes genitalis: _____

12. What clients are at risk of developing PIH?

_____

_____

_____

a. List the classic symptoms for PIH.

(1) _____

(2) _____

(3) _____

b. What are the three major goals of treatment for the client with PIH?

(1) _____

(2) _____

(3) _____

13. Chandra, a 21-year-old primigravida, is diagnosed with PIH. Because her symptoms are mild at present, she can remain at home. What will you tell Chandra about home management for PIH?

_____

_____

_____

a. What factors might lead to hospitalization for Chandra?

_____

_____

14. Mary Ann, a 23-year-old client, G1 P0, is O negative. Her husband is O positive. Will Mary Ann need RhoGAM during this pregnancy? If so, why?

_____

_____

_____

a. If this client is to receive RhoGAM, when would it be given?

_____

_____

_____

15. Belinda is a 24-year-old client with diabetes mellitus, type 1, diagnosed when she was a teenager. Her obstetric history includes two previous pregnancy losses, including a miscarriage last year. Belinda has poorly controlled diabetes as evidenced by high glucose levels and evidence of retinopathy. When asked, she admits she has not returned to her physician for diabetes management in "a long time." She is now approximately 10 weeks pregnant at her first prenatal visit. Belinda will be monitored closely for glucose levels and fetal well-being.

a. What effect will the pregnancy have on Belinda's diabetes?

_____

_____

_____

b. In what ways might her diabetes affect the pregnancy?

_____

_____

_____

c. What are the risks for the fetus related to Belinda's diabetes?

_____

_____

_____

d. Belinda tells you that she is very motivated to have a healthy baby with this pregnancy. What will she need to do to take care of herself while she is pregnant?

_____

_____

_____

e. How will the fetus be monitored during the pregnancy?

_____

_____

_____

f. How would preconception counseling have benefited Belinda?

_____

_____

_____

Self-Assessment Questions

Circle the letter that corresponds to the best answer.

1. You have been assigned to care for a client who is suspected of having HELLP syndrome as a result of PIH. You recall that this indicates your client may have all but which of the following complications?
   a. Hyperglycemia
   b. Lysing of red blood cells
   c. Decreased platelets
   d. Increased liver enzymes

2. The nurse is caring for a client with PIH who is receiving $MgSO_4$, a central nervous system depressant. To counteract respiratory depression that may occur with this medication, the nurse will be prepared to administer
   a. Narcan.
   b. Apresoline.
   c. epinephrine.
   d. calcium gluconate.

3. The nurse is caring for a client who is a 31-year-old multigravida diagnosed with gestational diabetes mellitus. Because of the effects of this disorder on the pregnancy, the nurse would anticipate a finding of
   a. macrosomia.
   b. hyporeflexia.
   c. oligohydramnios.
   d. peripheral edema.

4. The student is observing a fetal biophysical profile on her client, who is 35 weeks pregnant. The student recalls that this test should demonstrate fetal breathing and movement, fetal tone, amniotic fluid pockets, and
   a. a negative CST.
   b. a reactive NST.
   c. a negative Coombs' test.
   d. mild uterine contractions.

5. The nurse is caring for a client in active labor. The fetus is in a cephalic presentation at +2 station. With each contraction, the fetal heart rate is dropping after the acme of the contraction before returning to its baseline rate. The nurse determines that these are late decelerations caused by
   a. head compression.
   b. breech presentation.
   c. uteroplacental insufficiency.
   d. umbilical cord compression.

6. A nurse is performing an assessment on a client who is 33 weeks pregnant with a diagnosis of placenta previa. Which of the following findings will the nurse anticipate?
   a. Painless bleeding
   b. Abdominal rigidity
   c. Uterine tenderness
   d. Bright red bleeding

7. A general high-risk factor in pregnancy is that the client
   a. has diabetes.
   b. has had preeclampsia.
   c. has had a Cesarean birth.
   d. is unmarried.

8. The time of quickening is
   a. 8 to 12 weeks.
   b. 12 to 16 weeks.
   c. 16 to 20 weeks.
   d. 20 to 24 weeks.

9. When habitual abortions are caused by an incompetent cervix, it can be treated by
   a. a D&C.
   b. cerclage.
   c. a salpingectomy.
   d. induction of labor.

10. In an attempt to accelerate fetal lung maturity, a drug such as _____ may be given to the mother.
    a. betamethasone
    b. heparin
    c. methotrexate
    d. magnesium sulfate

The Birth Process

Key Terms

Match the following terms with their correct definitions.

___ 1. Acme

___ 2. Amniotomy

___ 3. Augmentation of labor

___ 4. Bloody Show

___ 5. Braxton-Hicks contractions

___ 6. Cephalopelvic disproportion

___ 7. Cervical dilation

___ 8. Cesarean birth

___ 9. Crowning

___10. Decrement

___11. Duration

___12. Dysfunctional labor

___13. Dystocia

___14. Effacement

a. Relationship of fetal body parts to one another, either flexion or extension.

b. Length of one contraction, from the beginning of the increment to the conclusion of the decrement.

c. Thin, fibrous membrane-covered space between skull bones.

d. Injection of a local anesthetic into the pudendal nerve to provide perineal, external genitalia, and lower vaginal anesthesia.

e. Condition in which the fetal head will not fit through the mother's pelvis.

f. Contractions that do not cause the cervix to dilate.

g. Unique ability of the muscle fibers of the uterus to remain shortened to a small degree after each contraction.

h. Labor with problems of the contractions or of maternal bearing down.

i. Expulsion of cervical secretions, blood-tinged mucus, and the mucous plug that blocked the cervix during pregnancy.

j. Relationship of the fetal presenting part to the ischial spines.

k. Relationship of the identified landmark on the presenting part to the four quadrants of the mother's pelvis.

l. Metal instruments used on the fetal head to provide traction or to provide a method of rotating the fetal head to an occiput-anterior position.

m. Condition of the umbilical cord being wrapped around the baby's neck.

n. Onset of regular contractions of the utuerus that cause cervical changes between 20 and 37 weeks' gestation.

____15. Engagement

____16. Episiotomy

____17. External version

____18. False labor

____19. Ferguson's reflex

____20. Fetal attitude

____21. Fetal lie

____22. Fetal position

____23. Fetal presentation

____24. Fontanelle

____25. Forceps

____26. Frequency

____27. Fundus

____28. Increment

____29. Induction of labor

____30. Intensity

____31. Interval

____32. Lightening

____33. Macrosomia

____34. Mechanism of labor

____35. Molding

____36. Nuchal cord

____37. Precipitate birth

____38. Precipitate labor

o. Long, difficult, or abnormal labor caused by any of the four major variables (4 P's) that affect labor.

p. Rotation of the fetal head back to be in normal alignment with the shoulders after delivery of the fetal head.

q. Incision in the perineum to facilitate passage of the baby.

r. Top of the uterus.

s. Medication that inhibits uterine contractions.

t. Peak of a contraction.

u. Stimulation of uterine contractions before contractions begin spontaneously for the purpose of birthing an infant.

v. Spontaneous, involuntary urge to bear down during labor.

w. Thinning of the cervix.

x. Artificial rupture of the membranes.

y. Irregular, intermittent contractions felt by the pregnant woman toward the end of pregnancy.

z. Manipulation of the fetus through the mother's abdomen to a presentation facilitating birth.

aa. Condition of the widest diameter of the fetal presenting part (head) entering the inlet to the true pelvis.

bb. Determined by the fetal lie and the part of the fetus that enters the pelvis first.

cc. Strength of the contraction at the acme.

dd. Enlargement of the cervical opening from 0 to 10 cm (complete dilation).

ee. Relationship of the cephalocaudal axis of the fetus to the cephalocaudal axis of the mother, either longitudinal or transverse.

ff. Increasing intensity of a contraction.

gg. Excessive fetal growth characterized by a fetus weighing more than 4,000 g (8.8 lb).

hh. Labor lasting less than 3 hours from the onset of contractions to the birth of the infant.

ii. Condition in which the umbilical cord lies below the presenting part of the fetus.

jj. Part of the fetus in contact with the cervix.

kk. Time from the beginning of one contraction to the beginning of the next contraction.

ll. Stimulation of uterine contractions after spontaneously beginning but having unsatisfactory progress of labor.

___39. Presenting part

mm. Birth of an infant through an incision in the abdomen and uterus.

___40. Preterm birth

nn. Membranous area where sutures meet on the fetal skull.

___41. Preterm labor

oo. When the largest diameter of the fetal head is past the vulva.

___42. Prolapsed cord

pp. Resting period between two contractions.

___43. Pudendal block

qq. Decreasing intensity of a contraction.

___44. Restitution

rr. Descent of the fetus into the pelvis, causing the uterus to tip forward, relieving pressure on the diaphragm.

___45. Station

ss. Birth occurring suddenly and unexpectedly without a CNM/physician present to assist.

___46. Suture

tt. Series of movements of the fetus as it passes through the pelvis and birth canal.

___47. Tocolytic agent

uu. Birth that takes place before the end of the 37th week of gestation.

___48. Uterine retraction

vv. Shaping of the fetal head to adapt to the mother's pelvis during labor.

Abbreviation Review

Write the meaning or definition of the following abbreviations and acronyms.

1. 4 P's _____
2. AROM _____
3. CNM _____
4. CPD _____
5. FHR _____
6. LDRP _____
7. LMA _____
8. LMP _____
9. LMT _____
10. LOA _____
11. LOP _____
12. LOT _____
13. LSA _____
14. LSP _____
15. LST _____
16. PROM _____
17. RMA _____
18. RMP _____
19. RMT _____
20. ROA _____

21. ROM _____

22. ROP _____

23. ROT _____

24. RSA _____

25. RSP _____

26. RST _____

27. SROM _____

28. VBAC _____

Exercises and Activities

1. Briefly describe how each of these four variables affects labor.

   Passage: _____

   _____

   Passenger: _____

   _____

   Powers: _____

   _____

   Psyche: _____

   _____

   a. How do nursing interventions support the psyche of a client in labor?

   _____

   _____

   _____

   b. List six signs of impending labor.

   (1) _____   (4) _____

   (2) _____   (5) _____

   (3) _____   (6) _____

   c. How do contractions differ in true versus false labor?

   _____

   _____

   d. What are the expected changes for each of the following during labor?

   Temperature: _____

   Pulse: _____

   Respirations: _____

   Blood pressure: _____

   White blood cell count: _____

   Gastrointestinal (GI) system: _____

2. For the following diagram, identify the fetal presentation, lie, attitude, and position. Draw an X over the place on the diagram where you would listen for the FHR.

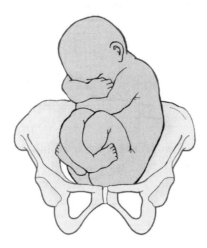

Fetal presentation _____

Fetal lie _____

Fetal attitude _____

Fetal position _____

3. Complete the following statements.
   a. The first stage of labor ends when the _____.
   b. The delivery of the placenta occurs at the end of the _____ stage of labor.
   c. A client is pushing during the _____ stage of labor.
   d. Transition is part of the _____ stage of labor.
   e. The shortest stage of labor is the _____ stage.
   f. The second stage of labor ends with the _____.

4. On the following graph, draw in the labor pattern using the descriptions given.

Frequency: 2 ½ minutes

Duration: 50 seconds

Intensity: moderate

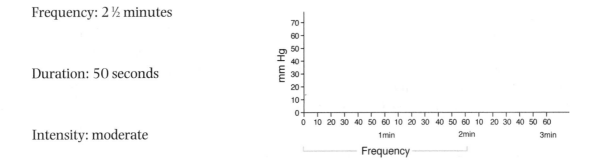

5. List two nursing interventions to support your client for each stage/phase of labor.

First stage:
Latent   1.
                2.

Active   1.
                2.

Transition	1.
	2.
Second stage	1.
	2.

6. Identify nursing interventions to support the mother and baby during the fourth stage of labor.

_____

_____

7. Using the following time lines, compare the length of each stage/phase of labor for the primigravida and the multigravida.

Primigravida	5 hr	10 hr	15 hr	20 hr	

Multigravida	5 hr	10 hr	15 hr	20 hr	

8. List risk factors for preterm labor.

   (1) _____

   (2) _____

   (3) _____

   (4) _____

   (5) _____

9. Susan and Jeffrey have just arrived at the birthing unit for the delivery of their first child. Susan is anxious and uncomfortable during her contractions. Jeffrey is excited about the birth and eager to help Susan. They attended all the childbirth classes but haven't been practicing the breathing and relaxation techniques. Describe nursing activities and interventions that can help Susan and Jeffrey to feel welcome and comfortable during admission.

   _____

   _____

   _____

   a. List questions you could ask Susan to obtain information about her labor.

   (1) _____

   (2) _____

   (3) _____

   (4) _____

   b. What information will be collected in the admission assessment?

   _____

   _____

c. What effect can Susan's anxiety have on her labor?

_____

_____

d. Susan needs support with her breathing techniques. How will you instruct Susan and Jeffrey in the first technique?

_____

_____

e. Susan had hoped for an unmedicated birth but is feeling overwhelmed with her contractions. A regional block is offered to her. List advantages and disadvantages of an epidural block for Susan.

Advantages	*Disadvantages*
_____	_____
_____	_____
_____	_____
_____	_____

10. Describe nursing actions for the immediate care of the newborn.

_____

_____

_____

_____

11. What are the five variables assessed with the Apgar score?

   (1) _____   (4)_____

   (2) _____   (5)_____

   (3) _____

12. If the birth involves the use of forceps or is vacuum assisted, how might the infant be affected?

_____

_____

_____

13. How can you promote maternal/infant bonding after delivery?

_____

_____

_____

14. Cynthia, a 29-year-old, G3 P2, arrives on the birthing unit early in the morning with her husband. She tells you that she was awakened this morning with a contraction. She tells you that she had short labors with her last delivery. Cynthia is full term and her pregnancy has been uneventful so far. Her membranes have ruptured. An assessment is completed and her physician has been notified.

a. Because Cynthia is in the active phase of labor, how often will you check her vital signs, FHR, and contractions?

_____

_____

_____

b. If Cynthia experiences a precipitate labor, what are the possible complications for her and the fetus?

_____

_____

c. Cynthia's labor is progressing well, but the FHR on the monitoring strip indicates that the fetal heart rate has dropped. Cynthia is advised she may have a Cesarean delivery. List several indications for a Cesarean birth.

(1) _____

(2) _____

(3) _____

(4) _____

(5) _____

(6) _____

d. What preoperative procedures and support will be initiated for Cynthia?

_____

_____

e. Following surgery with a horizontal uterine incision, the infant is suctioned, warmed, and assessed. Calculate the infant's Apgar score at 1 minute and 5 minutes.

	1 minute	5 minutes
Heart rate	96	126
Respiratory rate	Weak cry	Good cry
Muscle tone	Some flexion	Good flexion
Reflex irritability	Grimace	Crying
Color	Hands and feet blue	Body pink, extremities blue

Score

_____

f. The next day, Cynthia tells you she's just happy the baby is okay, but they had always hoped to have four children. Does this mean she has to have another cesarean birth if she gets pregnant again?

_____

_____

_____

_____

_____

_____

Self-Assessment Questions

Circle the letter that corresponds to the best answer.

1. The fetus of a laboring client is noted to be macrosomic. The nurse realizes that this may predispose this client to a longer, more difficult labor known as
   a. dystocia.
   b. hypertonia.
   c. uterine inertia.
   d. dysfunctional labor.

2. The nurse is caring for a laboring client who will be having an amniotomy. The first nursing action following this procedure will be to
   a. test the fluid with nitrazine paper.
   b. assess the fetal heart rate for 1 minute.
   c. assess the mother's vital signs and level of comfort.
   d. perform a vaginal exam to determine the dilation and effacement.

3. A client in labor is using breathing techniques to deal with the discomfort. The client is using slow, deep chest breathing, which is no longer effective to deal with the pain of her contractions. The nurse will advise this client to
   a. take Demoral IM.
   b. try pant-blow breathing.
   c. use relaxation techniques.
   d. advance to shallow breathing.

4. A nurse caring for a client in labor identifies a prolapsed cord occurring with the spontaneous rupture of membranes. Which of the following positions will the nurse utilize with this client?
   a. Supine
   b. Lithotomy
   c. Modified Sims'
   d. Reverse Trendelenburg

5. The risks to the fetus in a breech delivery include all but which of the following?
   a. Fluid aspiration
   b. Precipitate birth
   c. Cord compression
   d. Head becoming stuck

6. The nurse is monitoring oxytocin augmentation with a client whose membranes have ruptured but who has exhibited poor labor progress. For this client, the goal for oxytocin administration is to promote
   a. cervical ripening.
   b. hypotonic uterine contractions.
   c. contractions every 2 to 3 minutes, 45 to 60 seconds in length, of moderate intensity.
   d. contractions lasting 90 seconds with a uterine resting tone of at least 20 mm Hg.

7. When is labor induced after membrane rupture with a near-term pregnancy?
   a. 6–12 hours
   b. 12–24 hours
   c. 24–36 hours
   d. 36–48 hours

8. The position that improves labor progression is
   a. prone.
   b. supine.
   c. side-lying.
   d. dorsal recumbent.

9. The client is alert and talkative and the cervix is dilated 3 cm. The client is in the _____ phase.
   a. latent
   b. active
   c. transition
   d. focusing

10. Which mechanism of labor generally occurs during the first stage?
    a. Internal rotation
    b. Expulsion
    c. Extension
    d. Flexion

Postpartum Care

Key Terms

Match the following terms with their correct definitions.

___ 1. Afterpains	a. Term for the first 6 weeks after the birth of an infant.
___ 2. Attachment	b. Neurohormonal reflex that causes milk to be expressed from the alveoli into the lactiferous ducts.
___ 3. Bonding	c. Incomplete return of the uterus to its prepregnant size and consistency.
___ 4. Claiming process	d. Painful intercourse.
___ 5. Colostrum	e. Long-term process that begins during pregnancy and intensifies during the postpartum period that establishes an enduring bond between parent and child and develops through reciprocal (parent to child and child to parent) behaviors.
___ 6. Disseminated intravascular coagulation	f. Return of the reproductive organs, especially the uterus, to their prepregnancy size and condition.
___ 7. Dyspareunia	g. Uterine/vaginal discharge after childbirth; initially bright red, then changing to a pink or pinkish brown, then to a yellowish white.
___ 8. Engorgement	h. Newborn from birth to 28 days of life.
___ 9. Engrossment	i. Discomfort caused by the contracting uterus after the infant's birth.
___10. Entrainment	j. Infection following childbirth occurring between the birth and 6 weeks postpartum.
___11. Involution	k. Formation of a clot due to an inflammation in the wall of the vessel.
___12. Let-down reflex	l. Distention and swelling of the breasts in the first few days following delivery.
___13. Lochia	m. Abnormal stimulation of the clotting mechanism causing small clots throughout the vascular system and widespread bleeding internally, externally, or both.
___14. Mastitis	n. Rapid process of attachment, parent to infant, that takes place during the sensitive period, the first 30 to 60 minutes after the birth.

___15. Metritis

o. Inflammation of the fallopian tube.

___16. Neonate

p. Blood loss of more than 500 mL after the third stage of labor or 1,000 mL following a Cesarean birth.

___17. Oophoritis

q. Inflammation of the breast, generally during breast-feeding.

___18. Postpartum blues

r. Condition more severe than postpartum depression and characterized by delusions and thoughts of self-harm or infant harm.

___19. Postpartum depression

s. Process whereby a family identifies the infant's likeness to and differences from family members, and the infant's unique qualities.

___20. Postpartum hemorrhage

t. Inflammation of the ovary.

___21. Postpartum psychosis

u. Yellowish breast fluid rich in antibodies and high in protein.

___22. Puerperal (postpartum) infection

v. Mild transient condition of emotional liability and crying for no apparent reason, which affects up to 80% of women who have just given birth and lasts about 2 weeks.

___23. Puerperium

w. Parents' intense interest in and preoccupation with the newborn.

___24. Salpingitis

x. Inflammation of the uterus, including the endometrium and parametrium.

___25. Subinvolution

y. Infant's ability to move in rhythm to the parent's voice.

___26. Thrombophlebitis

z. Condition similar to postpartum blues but which is more serious, intense, and persistent.

Abbreviation Review

Write the meaning or definition of the following abbreviations, acronyms, and symbols.

1. CNM _____

2. DIC _____

3. DVT _____

4. hCG _____

5. hPL _____

6. MSH _____

7. PCA _____

8. PPD _____

9. RhoGAM _____

10. UTI _____

Exercises and Activities

1. How do the parents and family members establish attachment with the infant?

   _____

   _____

   _____

   a. What behaviors by the infant are important in bonding and attachment?

      _____

      _____

      _____

   b. Describe nursing actions and interventions that can facilitate bonding.

      _____

      _____

   c. Jackie expresses concern about how her 2-year-old daughter will react to the new baby. She does not feel they really prepared her for the birth. The daughter will be arriving with Dad in a little while. What guidance could you give Jackie?

      _____

      _____

      _____

      _____

      _____

2. Briefly describe physiological changes that occur during the postpartum period in each of the following.

   Uterus: _____

   _____

   Breasts: _____

   _____

   GI system: _____

   _____

   Urinary system: _____

   _____

   Musculoskeletal system: _____

   _____

   Blood values: _____

   _____

   a. What changes would the nurse anticipate in vital signs within the first 24 hours?

      _____

      _____

      _____

b. How do prolactin and oxytocin affect the postpartum client?

_____

_____

_____

c. Rebecca tells you that she will not need to use birth control for quite a while because she plans to breastfeed her newborn son for a year. What information would you share with her?

_____

_____

3. What are the main tasks for the mother in each phase of maternal restoration and adaptation according to Rubin?

Taking-in phase: _____

_____

Taking-hold phase: _____

_____

Letting-go phase: _____

_____

a. List several nursing actions or interventions that can facilitate the taking-hold phase.

(1) _____

(2) _____

(3) _____

(4) _____

(5) _____

(6) _____

b. Identify what each letter represents in the acronym BUBBLE for postpartum assessment.

B _____

U _____

B _____

B _____

L _____

E _____

c. What other subjective and objective information is collected during the assessment?

_____

_____

d. List factors that cause discomfort in the postpartum client.

_____

_____

e. Jeannie tells you during your assessment that she is having a lot of pain "in my bottom." What comfort measures can you offer or suggest?

_____

_____

_____

_____

4. How do postpartum blues differ from postpartum depression?

_____

_____

a. Identify factors that predispose the postpartum client to infection.

_____

_____

b. You are helping to discharge your client, Tracy, and her new baby today. The nurse asks you to review the signs and symptoms of postpartum infection with Tracy before she goes home. What information will you include?

_____

_____

5. Carla is a 17-year-old single mother, G1 P1, who has delivered an apparently healthy baby girl 3 hours ago with a Cesarean birth. Carla's mother is with her in the room and is holding the baby. She smiles and tells you this is their second grandchild. There is no information about the father of the baby. You notice that your client is very tired and is dozing on and off.

a. What additional assessment is necessary for Carla because she had a Cesarean birth?

_____

_____

_____

b. What special concerns may be related to Carla's age?

_____

_____

_____

c. After Carla has rested, you ask her if she would like to feed the baby. Carla tells you that she would like to try to breastfeed, but she does not have any milk yet. What will you tell her?

_____

_____

_____

_____

d. The next day, Carla has been encouraged to walk some and begin caring for herself and her baby. A few hours later, you notice Carla is still lying in bed. She tells you she is too tired and too uncomfortable to get up. Why is it important for her to become more active? How can you help Carla to balance her need for rest and activity?

_____

_____

_____

e. What observations might tell you whether Carla is adapting to her new role as mother?

_____

_____

_____

_____

_____

_____

Self-Assessment Questions

Circle the letter that corresponds to the best answer.

1. While assessing the postpartum client, the nurse makes the following findings. Which of these findings would *not* be expected during the first 24 hours after delivery?
   a. Diaphoresis
   b. Bradycardia
   c. Positive Homans' sign
   d. Temperature of 99.8°F

2. The nursing student is caring for a 39-year-old client who has given birth to her first baby. The student tells her instructor that the mother seems a little anxious and unsure of herself with her infant. She asks for help with infant care. The instructor reminds the student that this is
   a. typical behavior for an older mother.
   b. part of the taking-hold phase for the mother.
   c. a sign that the client is still in the taking-in phase.
   d. an indication of the mother's having a problem relating to her infant.

3. The nurse is assessing a postpartum client 2 days after delivery. The nurse notes that the fundus is firm, 2 cm below the umbilicus, she has lochia rubra with occasional small clots, and some edema of the perineum. The nurse will
   a. chart normal findings.
   b. medicate for uterine atony.
   c. note signs of puerperal infection.
   d. alert the CNM/physician to possible subinvolution.

4. The postpartum client is predisposed to urinary tract infection by all except which of the following factors?
   a. Urinary stasis after birth
   b. Trauma to the bladder and urethra
   c. Catheterization during labor or surgery
   d. Voiding every 2 hours after delivery

5. A new mother is breastfeeding her infant. At 3 days postpartum, she tells you her breasts are enlarged, warm, and tender. She also has a tingling or burning sensation in her nipples and a low-grade fever. The nurse advises the mother to
   a. use a breast pump to increase her comfort.
   b. discontinue breastfeeding and notify her CNM/physician.
   c. continue nursing the infant, because these are expected changes.
   d. supplement the infant with formula until her breasts return to normal size.

6. A behavior indicating that a toddler is adapting to a new infant in the home is:
   a. thumb sucking.
   b. bed wetting.
   c. hostility.
   d. independence.

7. The client's lochia is pinkish brown. This is called
   a. lochia rubra.
   b. lochia serosa.
   c. lochia alba.
   d. lochia drainage.

8. A laceration through the skin, mucous membrane, muscle, and rectal sphincter is considered
   _____ degree.
   a. first
   b. second
   c. third
   d. fourth

9. Oxytocin causes
   a. tingling and burning.
   b. milk expression.
   c. increased glucose levels.
   d. ovulation

10. A mother who cares lovingly for her infant but is unable to feel love is experiencing _____
    postpartum depression.
    a. mild
    b. moderate
    c. severe
    d. transient

Newborn Care

![black bar]

Key Terms

Match the following terms with their correct definitions.

___ 1. Acrocyanosis

___ 2. Appropriate for gestational age

___ 3. Caput succedaneum

___ 4. Cephalhematoma

___ 5. Circumcision

___ 6. Cold stress

___ 7. Conduction

___ 8. Convection

___ 9. Cryptorchidism

___10. Down syndrome

___11. Epispadias

___12. Epstein's pearls

___13. Erythema toxicum neonatorum

___14. Evaporation

___15. Foremilk

___16. Hallux varus

___17. Hindmilk

a. Maintenance of body temperature.

b. Whitish fluid secreted by a newborn's nipples.

c. Loss of heat when water is changed to a vapor.

d. Failure of one or both testes to descend.

e. First bowel movement of a newborn.

f. Saclike protrusion along the vertebral column filled with cerebrospinal fluid, meninges, nerve roots, and spinal cord.

g. Production of heat.

h. Environment in which the newborn can maintain internal body temperature with minimal oxygen consumption and metabolism.

i. Birthmark of enlarged superficial blood vessels, elevated and red in color.

j. Birthmarks of dilated capillaries that blanch with pressure; also called storkbites.

k. Infant's weight is above the 90th percentile for gestational age.

l. Metabolism of brown fat; process unique to the newborn.

m. White, creamy substance covering a fetus's body.

n. Infant's weight falls below the 10th percentile for gestational age.

o. Large reddish purple birthmark usually found on the face or neck that does not blanch with pressure.

p. Small, whitish yellow epithelial cysts found on the hard palate.

q. Edema of the newborn's scalp that is present at birth, may cross suture lines, and is caused by head compression against the cervix.

___18. Hydrocele

___19. Hyperbilirubinemia

___20. Hypospadias

___21. Kernicterus

___22. Lanugo

___23. Large for gestational age

___24. Meconium

___25. Meningocele

___26. Milia

___27. Molding

___28. Mongolian spots

___29. Myelomeningocele

___30. Neonatal transition

___31. Neutral thermal environment

___32. Nevus flammeus

___33. Nevus vascularis

___34. Nonshivering thermogenesis

___35. Ophthalmia neonatorum

___36. Phimosis

___37. Pseudomenstruation

___38. Radiation

r. Fine, downy hair covering the fetus's body.

s. Follows foremilk; is higher in fat content, leading to weight gain; and is more satisfying.

t. Blue coloring of hands and feet.

u. First few hours after birth wherein the newborn makes changes to and stabilizes respiratory and circulatory functions.

v. Collection of blood between the periosteum and the skull of a newborn; appears several hours to a day after birth, does not cross suture lines, and is caused by the rupturing of the periosteal bridging veins due to friction and pressure during labor and delivery.

w. Infant's weight falls between the 90th and 10th percentile for gestational age.

x. Placement of the great toe farther from the other toes.

y. Inflammation of the newborn's eyes that results from passing through the birth canal when a gonorrheal or chlamydial infection is present.

z. Congenital deformity in which the foot and ankle are twisted inward and cannot be moved to a midline position; also known as club foot.

aa. Saclike protrusion along the vertebral column filled with cerebrospinal fluid and meninges.

bb. Loss of heat by direct contact with a cooler object.

cc. Fluid around the testes in the scrotum.

dd. Surgical removal of the prepuce (foreskin) that covers the glans penis.

ee. Placement of the urinary meatus on the underside of the penis.

ff. Condition wherein the opening in the foreskin is so small that it cannot be pulled back over the glans.

gg. Loss of heat by transfer to cooler near objects, but not through direct contact.

hh. Excessive heat loss.

ii. Failure of the vertebral arch to close.

jj. Blood-tinged mucous discharge from the vagina of a newborn, caused by the withdrawal of maternal hormones.

kk. Watery first milk from the breast, high in lactose, like skim milk, and effective in quenching thirst.

ll. Loss of heat by the movement of air.

___39. Small for gestational age

___40. Spina bifida occulta

___41. Syndactyly

___42. Talipes equinovarus

___43. Telangiectactic nevi

___44. Thermogenesis

___45. Thermoregulation

___46. Vernix caseosa

___47. Witch's milk

mm. Pink rash with firm, yellow-white papules or pustules found on the chest, abdomen, back, and/or buttocks of a newborn.

nn. Excess of bilirubin in the blood.

oo. Severe neurological damage resulting from a high level of bilirubin (jaundice).

pp. Congenital chromosomal abnormality; also called trisomy 21.

qq. White, pinhead-size distended sebaceous glands on cheeks, nose, and chin.

rr. Fusion of two or more fingers or toes.

ss. Shaping of the fetal head to adapt to the mother's pelvis during labor.

tt. Large patches of bluish skin on the buttocks of dark-skinned infants.

uu. The placement of the urinary meatus on the top of the penis.

Abbreviation Review

Write the meaning or definition of the following abbreviations, acronyms, and symbols.

1. AAFP _____

2. AAP _____

3. ACIP _____

4. AGA _____

5. CPAP _____

6. FAS _____

7. HBIG _____

8. Hep B _____

9. IDM _____

10. ISAM _____

11. LGA _____

12. PKU _____

13. RDS _____

14. REM _____

15. SIDS _____

16. SGA _____

17. TTN _____

Exercises and Activities

1. List the four factors that help to initiate breathing in the newborn.

   (1) _____   (3) _____

   (2) _____   (4) _____

2. What four changes occur in the circulation of the newborn?

   _____

   _____

   _____

3. Describe how cold stress can lead to respiratory distress for the infant.

   _____

   _____

   _____

4. List the four methods of heat loss for the newborn and identify two interventions to prevent heat loss with each.

   (1)

          (1) _____

          (2) _____

   (2)

          (1) _____

          (2) _____

   (3)

          (1) _____

          (2) _____

   (4)

          (1) _____

          (2) _____

5. This was your first birth. "Congratulations!" you tell Amy and Matt after assisting with the difficult but rewarding vaginal birth of a baby boy. They have already named him Tyler, since they have known for some time it was going to be a boy. You are working today with Marsha, an experienced labor and delivery nurse who enjoys students. Marsha has already started taking care of Tyler's immediate needs after birth, including:

   (1) _____   (3) _____   (5) _____

   (2) _____   (4) _____   (6) _____.

   Marsha tells you, "We will be giving the baby an injection of vitamin K because:

   _____."

   "We also need to use erythromycin ointment because:

   _____

   _____."

a. You help Marsha by assessing Tyler's vital signs. They are, T—99.1°F; HR—154; R—62. Which are not in the normal range for vital signs? _____

b. Together, you and Marsha have completed Tyler's first physical assessment, noting all of the following findings. Circle those that could be due to the difficult delivery.

Acrocyanosis	Epstein's pearls	Edematous scrotum	Nevus vascularis
Cephalhematoma	Facial petechiae	Milia	Strabismus
Cryptorchidism	Flexed extremities	Molding	Subconjunctival hemorrhage
Ecchymosis	Lanugo	Mongolian spots	Telangiectatic nevi

c. Amy says, "Why is his head shaped so funny? Will it stay like that?" What will you tell the parents about molding?

_____

_____

d. You check Tyler's reflexes and demonstrate three of them for Matt and Amy. Describe how to elicit each of these reflexes:

Palmar grasp: _____

_____

Babinski's reflex: _____

_____

Moro reflex: _____

_____

Draw a line under the reflexes that will normally be gone by Tyler's 6-month checkup. Circle those that Tyler will need for breastfeeding.

Babinski's	Gallant	Placing	Sucking
Blinking	Hiccupping	Plantar grasp	Swallowing
Crossed extension	Moro	Rooting	Tonic neck
Extrusion	Palmar grasp	Stepping	Yawning

e. It is time to estimate Tyler's gestational age. You will be using the New Ballard Score for this, which you have found in your text. Marsha has already completed the neuromuscular maturity section for a score of 20. You offer to complete the physical maturity section. Draw an X on each block on the following scale that corresponds to the physical assessment findings.

	-1	0	1	2	3	4	5
Skin	sticky friable transparent	gelatinous red, translucent	smooth pink, visible veins	superficial peeling and or rash few veins	cracking pale areas rare veins	parchment deep cracking no vessels	feathery cracked wrinkled
Lanugo	none	sparse	abundant	thinning	bald areas	mostly bald	
Planiar Surface	heel-toe 40 - 50min: -1 <40 min: -2	>50mm no crease	faint red marks	anterior transverse crease only	creases ant. 2/3	creases over entire sole	
Breast	imperceptible	barely perceptible	flat areola no bud	stippled areola 1-2mm bud	raised areola 3-4mm bud	full areola 5-10mm bud	
Eye/Ear	lids fused loosely: -1 tightly: -2	lids open pinna flat stays folded	sl. curved pinna; soft slow recoil	well curved pinna; soft but ready recoil	formed and firm instant recoil	thick cartilage ear stiff	
Genitals Male	scrotum flat, smooth	scrotum empty faint rugae	testes in upper canal rare rugae	testes descending few rugae	testes down good rugae	testes pendulous deep rugae	
Genitals Female	clitoris prominant labia flat	prominant clitoris small labia minora	prominant clitoris enlarging minora	majora & minora equally prominant	majora large minora small	majora cover clitoris and minors	

He has some cracking on his skin, with rare veins.

Almost no lanugo remains.

Plantar creases cover the anterior two-thirds of the feet.

Breast tissue has a raised areola with a 4-mm bud.

The ears are formed and firm with instant recoil.

The testes are pendulous and have deep rugae.

Your total score for physical maturity is _____.

Added to Marsha's neuromuscular maturity score of 20, this gives a total of _____.

Using the Maturity Rating scale in Figure 54-19, what is his approximate gestational age based on this score? _____

Marsha says that comparing his weight, length, and head circumference, Tyler is AGA. What does this mean?

_____

_____

f. Your instructor stops by and says you can give the baby his first bath. Why is a thorough cleansing of the infant important? How will you maintain Tyler's temperature during the bath?

_____

_____

_____

g. You check on Amy and the baby a few hours later. Tyler is quietly gazing into his mother's eyes and has very little body movement. He seems to be watching and listening to his mother intently. You realize that Tyler is exhibiting a behavioral state called _____.

h. Amy and Matt are considering circumcision for their baby. If Tyler is circumcised, what are your nursing responsibilities?

_____

_____

_____

i. During a final visit the next day, you find Amy, Matt, and Tyler together. Amy is happy to see you because she needs some advice. The baby has been crying. Amy says that a relative told her she ought to start feeding the baby formula instead of breast milk because he sounds hungry all the time. You remind Amy that babies cry for other reasons, too, including:

_____

_____

You mention to Amy some of the advantages of breastfeeding, including:

(1) _____   (5) _____

(2) _____   (6) _____

(3) _____   (7) _____

(4) _____   (8) _____

j. Amy has a few more questions for you. Before you leave today, please go over them with her.

(1) "How often should Tyler breastfeed?"

(2) "How long should each feeding last?"

(3) "How can I tell if he is latched onto my breast properly?"

(4) "Since there is no 'air' in the breast, does Tyler need to be burped?"

(5) "How do I know if Tyler is getting enough milk?"

_____

_____

_____

_____

_____

Amy and Matt thank you for all your help. You have been so patient in answering all their questions. They are thinking of naming their next baby after you!

Self-Assessment Questions

Circle the letter that corresponds to the best answer.

1. A newborn has had difficulty maintaining its temperature within a normal range. The nurse recognizes that this can predispose the infant to
   a. cold stress.
   b. hyperglycemia.
   c. metabolic alkalosis.
   d. de-thermoregulation.

2. Which of the following physical assessment findings would the nurse observe in the preterm newborn with a gestational age of 35 weeks?
   a. Little or no lanugo
   b. Undescended testes
   c. Square window sign of 0°
   d. Creases on the anterior two-thirds of the sole

3. A nurse is caring for a new mother and infant. The nurse suspects transient tachypnea of the newborn because the infant is observed to have
   a. grade 0 on the Silverman-Anderson index.
   b. respiratory distress noted immediately after the birth.
   c. nasal flaring and a high respiratory rate several hours after birth.
   d. an irregular respiratory rate between 30 and 40 breaths per minute.

4. The nurse is caring for a new mother and infant after delivery. To facilitate mother–infant bonding and help initiate breastfeeding, the nurse will
   a. allow the infant to get hungry before beginning to breastfeed.
   b. leave the infant with its mother during the first period of reactivity.
   c. wait until the mother is fully rested after delivery to give her the infant.
   d. encourage mother–infant contact while the infant is in the active alert state.

5. The nursing instructor reminds the student to keep the newborn away from the cold window in the mother's room. This intervention will avoid heat loss in the newborn through
   a. radiation.
   b. convection.
   c. conduction.
   d. evaporation.

6. When an infant has nonshivering thermogenesis, it has:
   a. adequately raised its temperature.
   b. effectively increased its metabolism.
   c. now begun to metabolize brown fat.
   d. maintained heat retention.

7. A cold stethoscope is placed on an infant. The infant will have heat loss due to
   a. radiation.
   b. convection.
   c. conduction.
   d. evaporation.

8. A medication seldom used as an eye prophylaxis due to its lack of protection against chlamydial infection is:
   a. erythromycin.
   b. tetracycline.
   c. phytonadione.
   d. silver nitrate.

9. Bleeding from the cord is noted. The nurse should
   a. observe the cord bleeding for changes.
   b. check the clamp and apply a second clamp on the body side of the first one.
   c. clean the cord.
   d. check the clamp and apply a second clamp toward the outside of the first one.

10. Breast milk that has a higher fat content is called
    a. hindmilk.
    b. foremilk.
    c. colostrum.
    d. nutramigen.

Basics of Pediatric Care

Key Terms

Match the following terms with their correct definitions.

___ 1. Assent

___ 2. Child life specialist

___ 3. Emancipated minor

___ 4. Family-centered care

___ 5. Rooming-In

a. Health care professional with extensive knowledge of psychology and early childhood development.

b. Recognition that the family is the constant in a child's life, while the service systems and support personnel within those systems change (Shelton & Stepanek, 1994).

c. Voluntary agreement to participate in a research project or to accept treatment.

d. Practice of staying with the client 24 hours a day to provide care and comfort.

e. Child who has the legal competency of an adult because of circumstances involving marriage, divorce, parenting a child, living independently without parents, or enlistment in the armed services.

Abbreviation Review

Write the meaning or definition of the following abbreviations and acronyms.

1. BSA _____
2. DDST _____
3. EMLA _____
4. ID _____
5. IQ _____
6. NCHS _____
7. OBRA _____

Exercises and Activities

1. How does a child's developmental level affect the child's response to illness and health care?

   _____
   _____

2. Describe the nurse's role in supporting the child and family. Why are prevention and teaching important aspects of this role?

_____

_____

_____

3. List three factors or interventions that can help the family feel prepared for the hospitalization of a child.

(1) _____

(2) _____

(3) _____

4. How does rooming-in benefit the hospitalized child and family?

_____

_____

_____

5. Describe the role of a child life specialist in the health care setting.

_____

_____

_____

6. What measurements are assessed in the child under 2 years of age?

_____

_____

_____

7. What measurements are assessed in the child aged 2 years and older?

_____

_____

_____

8. Describe how to correctly assess the blood pressure of a child.

_____

_____

_____

9. Identify security measures used by health care agencies.

_____

_____

_____

10. You are caring for a young child who may need to have an extremity immobilized for several hours. What interventions might prevent the need for a restraint?

_____

_____

_____

11. If a restraint must be applied, what are your nursing responsibilities before and during its use? What documentation is needed?

_____

_____

_____

12. You are administering an oral medication to an infant. How would you proceed?

_____

_____

_____

13. List the advantages and disadvantages of IV medications.

_____

_____

_____

14. You are caring for a 7-year-old child with a terminal illness. Identify two interventions that may be helpful for each of the following:

      The child: (1)_____

                                    (2)_____

      Parents: (1)_____

                                      (2)_____

      Siblings: (1)_____

                                      (2)_____

   a. What support services might be helpful to the parents/family members?

_____

_____

   b. How can the nurse deal with personal feelings of grief?

_____

_____

15. Mariko is the 3-year-old daughter of Yuki and Ken Takeda. Mariko is scheduled to have heart surgery for the repair of an atrial septal defect (ASD) early next week. Other than concerns about the ASD, Mariko appears to be growing well and shows no developmental delays. She has not been hospitalized since birth. A quick recovery is anticipated.

   a. How can Mariko be prepared for the hospitalization and surgical experience?

_____

_____

   b. Although Yuki and Ken have anticipated the surgery for some time, they are now anxious and have many questions. What resources can be offered or suggested to help them feel more comfortable with the experience?

_____

_____

c. What information will the nurse collect at the time of admission?

_____

_____

d. How can the parents be incorporated into the care of their daughter?

_____

_____

e. List specific safety measures that the nurse would incorporate for this toddler.

_____

_____

f. What are the advantages of discharging Mariko home as soon as possible after the surgery?

_____

_____

_____

_____

_____

Self-Assessment Questions

Circle the letter that corresponds to the best answer.

1. The most important aspect for preparation of a child for hospitalization is
   a. preparation of the family.
   b. completing a developmental assessment.
   c. assigning a child life specialist to the care team.
   d. using age-specific books and pamphlets with the child.

2. The nurse is preparing medication to be administered to a young child. The most reliable method for determining the amount of medication to be used will be based on the child's
   a. age.
   b. weight.
   c. body surface area.
   d. degree of symptoms.

3. A nursing student is assisting in a well-baby clinic in the community. It is apparent that further instruction is needed when the student
   a. assesses the pulse apically for 1 full minute.
   b. compares the head and chest circumference in a 1-year-old.
   c. measures the height in the 1½-year-old in a recumbent position.
   d. measures the chest circumference 1 fingerbreadth below the nipple line.

4. The primary benefit of anxiety reduction for the child who is facing surgery is to reduce the
   a. anxiety of the parents.
   b. blood loss during surgery.
   c. preoperative medication needed.
   d. frequency of vital sign assessments.

5. A child is scheduled to have the Denver II performed. The parent asks the nurse what the purpose of this test is. The nurse responds by saying that the Denver II is a measurement tool that will determine
   a. whether any developmental delays exist.
   b. the child's IQ.
   c. how well the parent interacts with the child.
   d. whether the child's height and weight are within norms.

6. Federal guidelines state that children over 7 years of age have the right to give
   a. conscription.
   b. assent.
   c. informed consent.
   d. enlistment.

7. Normal vital signs for a 3-year-old could be
   a. temperature 98.8°F, pulse 160, respiratory rate 40, blood pressure 65/30.
   b. temperature 97.5°F, pulse 130, respiratory rate 36, blood pressure 70/46.
   c. temperature 97.5°F, pulse 120, respiratory rate 20, blood pressure 76/50.
   d. temperature 97.5°F, pulse 110, respiratory rate 14, blood pressure 90/60.

8. Normal vital signs for a 1 year old could be:
   a. temperature 98.8°F, pulse 160, respiratory rate 40, blood pressure 65/30.
   b. temperature 97.5°F, pulse 130, respiratory rate 36, blood pressure 70/46.
   c. temperature 97.5°F, pulse 120, respiratory rate 20, blood pressure 76/50.
   d. temperature 97.5°F, pulse 110, respiratory rate 14, blood pressure 90/60.

Infants with Special Needs: Birth to 12 Months

Key Terms

Match the following terms with their correct definitions.

___ 1. Abduction

a. Any intentional act of physical, emotional, or sexual abuse or neglect committed by a person responsible for the care of a child.

___ 2. Antipyretic

b. High-pitched, harsh sound heard on inspiration when the trachea or larynx is obstructed.

___ 3. Atresia

c. Surgical incision of the eardrum.

___ 4. Child abuse

d. Abnormal development.

___ 5. Circumoral cyanosis

e. Yellow discoloration of the skin, sclera, mucous membranes, and body fluids that occurs when the liver is unable to fully remove bilirubin from the blood.

___ 6. Colic

f. Lateral movement away from the body.

___ 7. Dislocation

g. Severe itching.

___ 8. Dysplasia

h. Displacement of a bone from its normal position in a joint.

___ 9. Erythematous

i. Impacted feces in the newborn, causing intestinal obstruction.

___10. Hypotonia

j. Large patches of bluish skin on the buttocks of dark-skinned infants.

___11. Intussusception

k. Forceful ejection (up to 3 feet) of the contents of the stomach.

___12. Jaundice

l. Lax muscle tone.

___13. Kernicterus

m. Saclike protrusion situated along the vertebral column and filled with spinal fluid, meninges, nerve roots, and spinal cord.

___14. Lecithin

n. Major component of surfactant.

___15. Meconium ileus

o. Telescoping of one part of the intestine into another.

___16. Meningitis

p. Drug used to reduce an abnormally high temperature.

___17. Milia

q. Characterized by reddishness of the skin.

___18. Mongolian spots

r. Condition of sudden, recurrent attacks of abdominal pain.

____19. Myelomeningocele

____20. Myringotomy

____21. Projectile vomiting

____22. Pruritus

____23. Stridor

s. Severe neurological damage resulting from a high level of bilirubin.

t. Absence or closure of a body orifice.

u. Bluish discoloration surrounding the mouth.

v. Pearly white cysts on the face.

w. Inflammation of the meninges.

Abbreviation Review

Write the meaning or definition of the following abbreviations and acronyms.

1. AGE _____

2. ASD _____

3. BPD _____

4. CF _____

5. CFTR _____

6. CHF _____

7. CNS _____

8. CP _____

9. CPAP _____

10. CPT _____

11. CSF _____

12. DDH _____

13. FTT _____

14. GER _____

15. GU _____

16. LTB _____

17. NGT _____

18. PDA _____

19. PMI _____

20. RDS _____

21. RSV _____

22. SCA _____

23. SIDS _____

24. TOF _____

25. UTI _____

26. VSD _____

27. WIC _____

Exercises and Activities

1. Why is it important to understand the differences in the systems of the infant versus the adult?

   _____

   _____

   _____

2. List differences in the respiratory tract of the infant that increase the risk for obstruction and aspiration.

   _____

   _____

   _____

3. Describe the signs and symptoms of pneumonia that might be noted in the infant.

   _____

   _____

   _____

4. List several nursing interventions for the infant with pneumonia.

   (1) _____   (4) _____

   (2) _____   (5) _____

   (3) _____   (6) _____

5. Describe signs and symptoms of respiratory distress syndrome.

   _____

   _____

   _____

6. How would you explain the cause of cystic fibrosis to the parents of an infant with this disorder? What symptoms would the infant or child experience?

   _____

   _____

   _____

7. Leah has just been diagnosed with her second ear infection in 3 months. What causes an infant to be susceptible to otitis media? What signs and symptoms should her parents watch for that would indicate an infection?

   _____

   _____

   _____

8. What differences in the gastrointestinal (GI) system in infants increase their risk for GI disorders?

   (1) _____   (5) _____

   (2) _____   (6) _____

   (3) _____   (7) _____

   (4) _____

9. You are assessing for signs of dehydration in an infant with a GI disorder. What signs and symptoms would you note?

_____

_____

_____

10. How can fluid intake be encouraged in the infant who is at risk of dehydration?

_____

_____

_____

11. Matthew's mother tells you during her baby's 6-week checkup that he seems unusually colicky. She realizes that new babies cry a lot, but Matthew just cries for hours at a time. Nothing she does seems to help. What questions will you ask Matthew's mother? What suggestions can you give that may alleviate his colic?

_____

_____

_____

12. Jeremy is being assessed at the pediatric clinic 2 days after his birth for his first well-baby visit. A right-sided hip click was noted at birth. What other findings might indicate hip dislocation? What would treatment for Jeremy include?

_____

_____

_____

13. What are signs of physical neglect and abuse in an infant?

_____

_____

_____

14. List several safety measures that are appropriate for the child's first year of life.

_____

_____

_____

_____

15. You are caring for Alexis, the new daughter of John and Caroline Taylor. Alexis is a full-term infant weighing 7 lb, 8 oz and is 19 in. in length. However, Alexis was born with a cleft lip on the left side and a cleft palate. Although Caroline and John are thrilled to be parents, they are visibly distressed about this congenital defect. They wonder how she will eat, how they will care for her, and when her lip and mouth can be repaired.

a. How will you support John and Caroline following the birth of their infant?

_____

_____

b. Why is an interdisciplinary approach important to Alexis's care?

_____

_____

c. Identify complications that Alexis is at risk for before her surgical repair.

_____

_____

d. Caroline asks you to help her feed Alexis with a special bottle and nipple. What suggestions will you make to help with the feeding?

_____

_____

e. When will the infant's cleft lip and palate be repaired?

_____

_____

f. List nursing interventions that will promote healing following the repair of her cleft palate.

(1) _____   (4) _____

(2) _____   (5) _____

(3) _____   (6) _____

Self-Assessment Questions

Circle the letter that corresponds to the best answer.

1. The newborn who has a history of frank breech position, is large for gestational age, or is a twin is at greater risk for
   a. club foot.
   b. hypotonia.
   c. hip dysplasia.
   d. developmental delays.

2. A 10-month-old child is recovering from a sickle-cell crisis. To prevent a recurrence of a sickle-cell crisis for this child, the nurse encourages the parents to do all but which of the following?
   a. Delay immunizations.
   b. Avoid cold temperatures.
   c. Use prophylactic antibiotics.
   d. Maintain adequate hydration.

3. A 1-year-old has just experienced a febrile seizure. The nurse emphasizes to the parents that febrile seizures
   a. usually last for several minutes.
   b. do not cause neurological sequelae.
   c. increase the risk of seizure disorder in childhood.
   d. can be prevented by prompt administration of aspirin for fever.

4. When caring for an infant with acute gastroenteritis, it is most important for the nurse to assess the infant for
   a. dehydration.
   b. abdominal pain.
   c. intake and output.
   d. number of diarrheal stools.

5. An infant arrives at the community clinic with signs of an upper respiratory illness. The infant has mild stridor when active, a barking cough, and hoarseness. The temperature is 99.6°F, and there is a nasal discharge. It is most important to instruct the parents to
   a. increase fluid intake.
   b. maintain a humid environment.
   c. watch for signs of respiratory distress.
   d. suction the mouth and nose for mucus.

6. What is *not* considered a clinical manifestation of abuse?
   a. Bruises on the abdomen
   b. Multiple bone fractures at various stages of healing
   c. Withdrawal
   d. Mongolian spots

7. A clinical manifestation present in ventricular septal defect is
   a. delayed growth and development.
   b. dysrhythmias.
   c. increased respiratory infections.
   d. a machine-like murmur.

8. A clinical manifestation present in tetralogy of fallot is
   a. delayed growth and development.
   b. dysrhythmia.
   c. increased respiratory infection.
   d. a machine-like murmur.

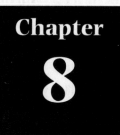

Common Problems: 1–18 Years

Chapter 8

Key Terms

Match the following terms with their correct definitions.

___ 1. Acanthesis nigricans

___ 2. Comedone

___ 3. Encopresis

___ 4. Epistaxis

___ 5. Gowers' Sign

___ 6. Rhinorrhea

a. Watery nasal discharge.

b. Passage of watery colonic contents around a hard fecal mass.

c. Whitehead or blackhead.

d. Hemorrhage of the nares or nostrils; also known as nosebleed.

e. Walking the hands up the legs to get from a sitting to a standing position (as in Duchenne muscular dystrophy).

f. A velvety hyperpigmented patch on the back of the neck, axilla, or antecubital area.

Abbreviation Review

Write the meaning or definition of the following abbreviations and acronyms.

1. AAP _____

2. ACIP _____

3. ADHD _____

4. ALL _____

5. APSGN _____

6. ASO _____

7. BMI _____

8. CPT _____

9. DMD _____

10. DTaP _____

11. ER _____

12. ESR _____

13. FPG _____

14. HBV _____

15. HSV _____

16. IPV _____

17. ITP _____

18. JA _____

19. MCNS _____

20. MDI _____

21. MMR _____

22. OPV _____

23. PCOS _____

24. RAD _____

25. TIG _____

Exercises and Activities

1. What factors put children at greater risk for parasitic infections than adults?

   _____

   _____

   _____

2. How would you differentiate pharyngitis from influenza? Are there differences in the treatment?

   _____

   _____

   _____

3. What are early signs and symptoms of asthma? What assessment findings might be noted in children with chronic asthma?

   _____

   _____

   _____

4. Jamal, a 6-year-old boy in your pediatric clinic, has been recently diagnosed with asthma. What information will you give to Jamal's parents about ways to manage his asthma at home?

   _____

   _____

   _____

5. Describe the pharmacological treatment for asthma.

   _____

   _____

   _____

6. List signs and symptoms and the medical–nursing management for each of the following common pediatric disorders.

	Signs and Symptoms	Treatment
Impetigo		
Pediculosis		
Acne		

7. How would you detect scoliosis during a routine screening of adolescents?

_____

_____

_____

8. Describe symptoms that might be noted in a child with ADHD. What are the goals for nursing care for a child with ADHD?

_____

_____

_____

9. Identify several risk factors for suicide.

(1) _____   (5) _____

(2) _____   (6) _____

(3) _____   (7) _____

(4) _____   (8) _____

10. What behaviors might indicate to you that an individual is considering suicide?

_____

_____

_____

11. Of the following communicable diseases, underline those for which there is a vaccine. Circle those that are transmitted by way of respiratory droplets.

Chickenpox	Hepatitis B	Mumps	Roseola
Diphtheria	Measles	Pertussis	Rubella
Fifth disease	Mononucleosis	Poliomyelitis	Scarlet fever
			Tetanus

12. Identify four barriers to immunization.

(1) _____   (3) _____

(2) _____   (4) _____

13. The mother of a newborn tells you that she is concerned about having her baby immunized. She has heard that some immunizations can have serious side effects and cause long-term complications. What would you tell her?

_____

_____

_____

14. What is the nurse's responsibility related to immunizations and documentation?

_____

_____

_____

15. Daniel, who is 9 years old, was brought in to the pediatric office by his mother. She tells you that he had a fever at home of 101°F, pain in his joints, and a pinkish rash. During the health history, his mother reveals that Daniel had an untreated upper respiratory infection with a bad sore throat about a month ago. He seemed to get over it at the time without too much trouble. Daniel is now suspected of having rheumatic fever.

a. List laboratory test results that might confirm this diagnosis.

_____

_____

b. What other signs and symptoms might Daniel exhibit with rheumatic fever?

_____

_____

c. Identify the goals of medical management.

(1) _____

(2) _____

(3) _____

d. What will Daniel's treatment include?

_____

_____

_____

e. List long-term complications that can result from rheumatic fever.

_____

_____

_____

f. Daniel's mother wants to know if he can ever get rheumatic fever again. What will you tell her?

_____

_____

_____

Self-Assessment Questions

Circle the letter that corresponds to the best answer for each question.

1. The nurse is caring for a child diagnosed with asthma. To reduce mucosal edema and improve the effect of a bronchodilator, the physician orders
   a. Alupent.
   b. Brethine.
   c. prednisone.
   d. theophylline.

2. Laboratory test results show that a young child has ITP. The nurse recalls that ITP is
   a. most common in school-aged children.
   b. cured with antibiotics if diagnosed early.
   c. a complication of a streptococcus infection.
   d. an autoimmune disorder that destroys platelets.

3. The nurse is performing an assessment on a child who is ill with rheumatic fever. All but which of the following findings might the nurse anticipate?
   a. Chorea
   b. Polyarthritis
   c. Strawberry tongue
   d. Subcutaneous nodules

4. A child with fever, headache, sore throat, and rash has just been diagnosed with scarlet fever. You explain to the parents that their child
   a. will be treated with penicillin.
   b. will have lifelong immunity after recovery.
   c. may have complications such as meningitis.
   d. is not contagious after symptoms have begun.

5. Home treatment for asthma may include all but which of the following interventions?
   a. Family education
   b. Chest physiotherapy
   c. Use of a peak flowmeter
   d. Restriction of physical activity

6. An elevated _____ is indicative of a recent streptococcal infection.
   a. ASO
   b. ESR
   c. C-reactive protein
   d. leukocyte

7. Mild hemophilia may
   a. be detected from bleeding from the umbilical cord.
   b. not be detected until a toddler becomes mobile.
   c. not ever show any clinical manifestations.
   d. be detected from bleeding from a circumcision site.

8. Itching around the anus may indicate which common intestinal parasite?
    a. Giardiasis
    b. Roundworm
    c. Pinworm
    d. Hookworm

Answer Key

Chapter 1   Prenatal Care

Key Terms

1. j
2. d
3. i
4. t
5. l
6. f
7. gg
8. aa
9. cc
10. m
11. z
12. c
13. tt
14. u
15. aaa
16. dd
17. fff
18. g
19. qq
20. bbb
21. v
22. ll
23. ccc
24. vv
25. yy
26. ee
27. xx
28. ss
29. uu
30. kk
31. mm
32. n
33. ggg
34. pp
35. rr
36. ddd
37. ww
38. eee
39. zz
40. hh
41. o
42. ii
43. p
44. y
45. a
46. r
47. w
48. b
49. bb
50. ff
51. jj
52. s
53. nn
54. e
55. h
56. oo
57. k
58. x
59. q

Abbreviation Review

1. American Society for Psychoprophylaxis in Obstetrics
2. Association of Women's Health, Obstetric, and Neonatal Nurses
3. bag of water
4. biparietal diameter
5. crown-heel
6. crown-rump
7. diethylstilbestrol
8. estimated date of birth
9. estimated date of delivery
10. gravida, para/term, preterm, abortions, living
11. glomerular filtration rate
12. human chorionic gonadotropin
13. Fetal hemoglobin

14. human placental lactogen
15. International Childbirth Education Association
16. last menstrual period
17. Nurses Association of the American College of Obstetricians and Gynecologists
18. over-the-counter
19. protein bound iodine

Self-Assessment Questions

1. a
2. d
3. c
4. b
5. d
6. a
7. a
8. d
9. b
10. d

Chapter 2   Complications of Pregnancy

Key Terms

1. d
2. l
3. e
4. h
5. m
6. a
7. k
8. c
9. n
10. f
11. r
12. p
13. s
14. u
15. b
16. i
17. o
18. g
19. q
20. t

21. v
22. j

Abbreviation Review

1. cytomegalovirus
2. contraction stress test
3. chorionic villi sampling
4. dilatation and curettage
5. disseminated intravascular coagulation
6. estimated date of birth
7. electronic fetal monitoring
8. fetal acoustic stimulation test
9. fetal biophysical profile
10. fetal heart rate
11. fetal heart tones
12. gestational diabetes mellitus
13. human chorionic gonadotrophin
14. hemolysis, elevated liver enzymes, low platelet count
15. human placental lactogen
16. herpes simplex virus type 2
17. intrauterine growth retardation
18. lecithin/sphingomyelin
19. magnesium sulfate
20. maternal serum alpha-fetoprotein
21. nonstress test
22. phosphatidyglycerol
23. pregnancy-induced hypertension
24. phenylketonuria
25. Rh immune globulin
26. small for gestational age
27. toxoplasmosis, rubella, cytomegalovirus, herpes virus type 2
28. vibroacoustic stimulation test

Self-Assessment Questions

1. a
2. d
3. a
4. b
5. c
6. a
7. d
8. c
9. b
10. a

Chapter 3 The Birth Process

Key Terms

1. t
2. x
3. ll
4. i
5. y
6. e
7. dd
8. mm
9. oo
10. qq
11. b
12. h
13. o
14. w
15. aa
16. q
17. z
18. f
19. v
20. a
21. ee
22. k
23. bb
24. nn
25. l
26. kk
27. r
28. ff
29. u
30. cc
31. pp
32. rr
33. gg
34. tt
35. vv
36. m
37. ss
38. hh
39. jj
40. uu
41. n
42. ii
43. d
44. p
45. j
46. c
47. s
48. g

Abbreviation Review

1. passage, passenger, powers, pysche
2. artificial rupture of membranes
3. certified nurse midwife
4. cephalopelvic disproportion
5. fetal heart rate
6. labor, delivery, recovery, postpartum
7. left mentum anterior
8. left mentum posterior
9. left mentum transverse
10. left occiput anterior
11. left occiput posterior
12. left occiput transverse
13. left sacrum anterior
14. left sacrum posterior
15. left sacrum transverse
16. premature rupture of membranes
17. right mentum anterior
18. right mentum posterior
19. right mentum transverse
20. right occiput anterior
21. rupture of membranes
22. right occiput posterior
23. right occiput transverse
24. right sacrum anterior
25. right sacrum posterior
26. right sacrum transverse
27. spontaneous rupture of membranes
28. vaginal birth after cesarean

Self-Assessment Questions

1. a
2. b
3. d
4. c
5. b
6. c
7. b
8. c
9. a
10. d

Chapter 4   Postpartum Care

Key Terms

1. i
2. e
3. n
4. s
5. u
6. m
7. d
8. l
9. w
10. y
11. f
12. b
13. g
14. q
15. x
16. h
17. t
18. v
19. z
20. p
21. r
22. j
23. a
24. o
25. c
26. k

Abbreviation Review

1. breasts, uterus, bladder, bowel, lochia, and episiotomy
2. certified nurse midwife
3. disseminated intravascular coagulation
4. deep vein thrombosis
5. human chorionic gonadotropin
6. human placental lactogen
7. melanocyte-stimulating hormone
8. patient-controlled analgesia
9. postpartum depression
10. Rh immune globulin
11. urinary tract infection

Self-Assessment Questions

1. c
2. b
3. a
4. d
5. c
6. d
7. b
8. c
9. b
10. a

Chapter 5   Newborn Care

Key Terms

1. t
2. w
3. q
4. v
5. dd
6. hh
7. bb
8. ll
9. d
10. pp
11. uu
12. p
13. mm
14. c
15. kk
16. x
17. s
18. cc
19. nn
20. ee
21. oo
22. r
23. k
24. e
25. aa
26. qq
27. ss
28. tt
29. f
30. u
31. h
32. o
33. i
34. l

35. y
36. ff
37. jj
38. gg
39. n
40. ii
41. rr
42. z
43. j
44. g
45. a
46. m
47. b

Abbreviation Review

1. American Academy of Family Physicians
2. American Academy of Pediatrics
3. Advisory Committee on Immunization Practices
4. appropriate for gestational age
5. continuous positive airway pressure
6. fetal alcohol syndrome
7. hepatitis B immune globulin
8. hepatitis B
9. infant of a diabetic mother
10. infant of a substance abusing mother
11. large for gestational age
12. phenylketonuria
13. respiratory distress syndrome
14. rapid eye movement
15. sudden infant death syndrome
16. small for gestational age
17. transient tachypnea of the newborn

Self-Assessment Questions

1. a
2. b
3. c
4. b
5. a
6. c
7. c
8. d
9. b
10. a

Chapter 6   Basics of Pediatric Care
Key Terms

1. c
2. a
3. e
4. b
5. d

Abbreviation Review

1. body surface area
2. Denver Developmental Screening Test
3. eutectic (cream) mixture of local anesthetics
4. identification
5. intelligence quotient
6. National Center for Health Statistics
7. Omnibus Budget Reconciliation Act

Self-Assessment Questions

1. a
2. b
3. d
4. c
5. a
6. b
7. c
8. b

Chapter 7   Infants with Special Needs: Birth to 12 Months
Key Terms

1. f
2. p
3. t
4. a
5. u
6. r
7. h
8. d
9. q
10. l
11. o
12. e
13. s
14. n
15. i
16. w

17. v
18. j
19. m
20. c
21. k
22. g
23. b

Abbreviation Review

1. acute gastroenteritis
2. atrial septal defect
3. bronchopulmonary dysplasia
4. cystic fibrosis
5. cystic fibrosis transmembrane regulator
6. congestive heart failure
7. central nervous system
8. cerebral palsy
9. continuous positive airway pressure
10. chest physiotherapy
11. cerebrospinal fluid
12. developmental dysplasia of the hip
13. failure to thrive
14. gastroesophageal reflux
15. genitourinary
16. laryngotracheobronchitis
17. nasogastric tube
18. patent ductus arteriosis
19. point of maximum intensity
20. respiratory distress syndrome
21. respiratory syncytial virus
22. sickle-cell anemia
23. sudden infant death syndrome
24. tetralogy of Fallot
25. urinary tract infection
26. ventricular septal defect
27. Women, Infants, and Children

Self-Assessment Questions

1. c
2. a
3. b
4. a
5. c
6. d
7. c
8. a

Chapter 8   Common Problems: 1–18 Years

Key Terms

1. f
2. c
3. b
4. d
5. e
6. a

Abbreviation Review

1. American Academy of Pediatrics
2. Advisory Committee on Immunization Practices
3. attention deficit hyperactivity disorder
4. acute lymphocytic leukemia
5. acute poststreptococcal glomerulonephritis
6. antistreptolysin-O
7. body mass index
8. chest physiotherapy
9. Duchenne muscular dystrophy
10. diphtheria, tetanus, acellular pertussis
11. emergency room
12. erythrocyte sedimentation rate
13. fasting plasma glucose
14. hepatitis B virus
15. herpes simplex virus
16. inactivated polio vaccine
17. idiopathic thrombocytopenic purpura
18. juvenile arthritis
19. minimal change nephrotic syndrome
20. metered-dose inhaler
21. measles, mumps, rubella
22. oral polio vaccine
23. polycystic ovarian syndrome
24. reactive airway disease
25. tetanus immune globulin

Self-Assessment Questions

1. c
2. d
3. c
4. a
5. d
6. a
7. b
8. c